HOLISM
AND BEYOND

The Essence of Holistic Medicine

Two Perspectives

Other Books by Dr. John Diamond:

Your Body Doesn't Lie

*Life Energy: Unlocking the Hidden Power of Your
    Emotions to Achieve Total Well-Being*

Life-Energy Analysis: A Way to Cantillation

The Re-Mothering Experience: How to Totally Love

The Life Energy in Music (The Life Energy in Music, Vol. I)

The Wellspring of Music (The Life Energy in Music, Vol. II)

The Heart of Music (The Life Energy in Music, Vol. III)

A Spiritual Basis of Holistic Therapy

The Collected Papers, Volumes I and II

Speech, Language and the Power of the Breath

A Book of Cantillatory Poems

The Healer: Heart and Hearth

The Healing Power of Blake: A Distillation

The Way of the Pulse: Drumming with Spirit

Life Enhancement Through Music

The Veneration of Life: Through the Disease to the Soul

Music and Song, Mother and Love

HOLISM AND BEYOND

The Essence of Holistic Medicine

Two Perspectives

John Diamond, M.D.

**D.P.M., F.R.A.N.Z.C.P., M.R.C. Psych.,
F.I.A.P.M., D.I.B.A.K.**

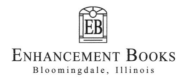

ENHANCEMENT BOOKS
Bloomingdale, Illinois

HOLISM AND BEYOND:
The Essence of Holistic Medicine

First published and printed in 2001.

Copyright ©2001 by John Diamond, M.D.
All rights reserved.

Cover photograph by John Diamond

Published by: Enhancement Books
               PO Box 544
               Bloomingdale, IL 60108
               USA
               Web: www.vitalhealth.net
               E-mail: vitalhealth@compuserve.com

Printed in the United States of America

ISBN 1-890995-37-1

In loving memory of

Dr. Robert Fulford
Dr. Ainslie Meares
Dr. Hans Nieper

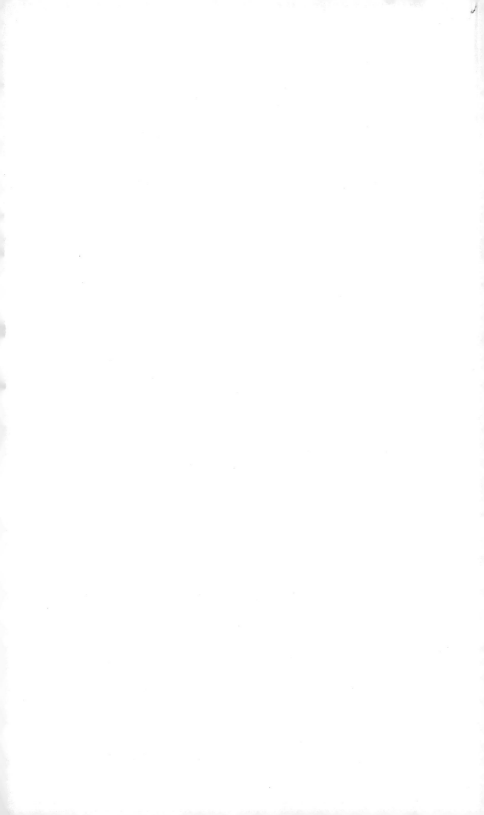

The Wholistic Universe

I saw eternity the other night
Like a great ring of pure and endless light,
All calm as it was bright.

HENRY VAUGHN

Let us start by considering the origin of the word *holism*. When you consult the *Oxford English Dictionary* you make a surprising discovery. Holism is a very new word. It has only been in recorded existence since 1926, being coined by a remarkable man, Jan Christian Smuts. Smuts knew his etymology and, in fact checked out the correctness of the word with the great Greek scholar, Gilbert Murray. Here is the *Oxford English Dictionary* definition of holism:

> *A term coined by Gen. J.C. Smuts (1870–1950) to designate the tendency in nature to produce wholes (i.e. bodies or organisms) from the ordered grouping of unit structures. . . . The whole-making holistic tendency, or Holism, operating in and through particular wholes, is seen at all stages of existence.*

The first recorded usage in medicine is not until 1960 – by F. H. Hoffman in *Psychosomatics*:

> *Throughout the United States, concern with teaching about the whole man – 'holistic' or comprehensive medicine – is*

a growing phenomenon in the medical school curriculum. [If only that were true!]

Smuts wrote it without the *w* – holistic. Some quibble with this, relating it of course to the word whole. But the *w* in whole is an affectation which came into English during the fifteenth or sixteenth century. Later, when we consider the etymology, you will see that his spelling is indeed correct.

Smuts was twice Prime Minister of South Africa. He was one of the leading figures in the foundation of the League of Nations and one of the very first statesmen to visit defeated Germany after the war as an act of reconciliation. He wrote his seminal book in 1926 called *Holism and Evolution,* in a period when he was out of power. Among other things, he understood what was then called the new physics. He is said to have given an explanation of Einstein's Theory of Relativity which was so easy to understand that people doubted that it could be valid.

One of the seminal writers in Smuts's life, who helped him with his concept of holism, was Walt Whitman: "every atom belonging to me as good belongs to you." (Whitman's influence has been enormous, extending to Gandhi, and including two of his physicians, both concerned with holism: William Osler and Richard Bucke [*Cosmic Consciousness*].)

The *Random House Dictionary* defines *holism* as "the theory that whole entities, as fundamental components of reality, have an existence other than as the mere sum of their parts."

And the *Encyclopedia Britannia* describes it as:

> *The philosophical theory based on the presuppositions of emergent evolution, that entirely new things – 'wholes' – are produced by a creative force within the universe; they are consequently more than mere arrangements of particles that already existed.*

Thus there are wholes and there is a process of holism to create wholes. This concept was taken up very quickly and widely. The *Cambridge Dictionary of Philosophy* defines it as: "Any of a wide variety of theses that in one way or another affirm the equal or greater reality, or the explanatory necessity of the whole of some system in relation to its parts." It then lists metaphysical holism, methodological holism, semantic holism, doxastic holism, epistemic holism, and so forth.

So the concept of holism became very widespread, with little credit being given to Smuts, and with many applications sharing very little understanding of what he was really trying to say: that there is a creative force toward the construction of wholes which are greater than the sum of their parts. And this applies from atomic physics all the way to cosmology. Including, of course, holistic medicine.

Bertrand Russell writes that there are really two schools of philosophy: the analysis and the synthesis. Those that break things down into little bits, and those like Smuts who try to create wholes. Breaking into bits, cutting people into pieces, is much easier than seeing them holistically. But, you don't learn holism from dissection.

As Russell says:

> [This] *is the question that divides the friends of analysis from its enemies... Suppose I say 'John is the father of James.' Hegel, and all who believe in what Marshal Smuts calls 'holism' will say: 'Before you can understand this statement, you must know who John and James are.' Now to know who John is, is to know all his characteristics, for apart from them he would not be distinguishable from anyone else. But all his characteristics involve other people or things. He is characterized by his relations to his parents, his wife, his children, by whether he is a good or a bad citizen, and by the country to which he belongs. All these things you must know before you can be said to know whom the word 'John' refers to.*[1]

This – and more – is what I call the holistic medical conception. If we're going to examine a

---

[1] *A History of Western Philosophy*. New York: Simon & Schuster, 1972.

sufferer holistically we need to know all of this and more. Who is the patient? Who is John? Russell continues:

Step by step, in your endeavour to say what you mean by the word 'John,' you will be led to take account of the whole universe, and your original statement will turn out to be telling you something about the universe, not about two separate people, John, and James.

But it will tell you also of John and James. Russell failed to recognize that John and James were merely parts of the whole. He was a philosopher only of the mind – that was his limitation.

For the end-point of knowledge is heart-Knowledge: All is One, All is Love. All is One is Love.

Pico Della Mirandola (1463–1494), a philosopher not of the brain but of the heart wrote:

We prefer constantly to seek through knowledge [that is, analysis], *never finding what we seek, rather than to possess through love that which without love would be found in vain.*[2]

The path to holism starts with the desire to love and ends with finding it.

---

[2] Mirandola, Pico Della. *Of Being and Unity*, trans. V. Hamm. Milwaukee: Marquette University Press, 1943.

John Dewey sought not only brain-knowledge but also heart-knowledge – to really Know:

To assume that anything can be known in isolation from its connections with other things is to lose the key to the traits that distinguish an object as known. . . . The more connections and interactions we ascertain, the more we know the object in question.[3]

So again he is concerned with building up a total *whole* picture of the person in his *whole* existence. *This is the only way to Know.* This is what I believe about holistic medicine.

To make the following quote from Hegel more apposite here, we can replace what he calls the "Idea" with "the whole" or "holism":

Each of the parts of philosophy is a philosophical whole, a circle rounded and complete in itself. In each of these parts, however, the philosophical Idea is found in a particular specificity or medium. The individual circle, since it is internally a totality, bursts through the limits imposed by its special medium, and gives rise to a wider circle. The whole thus resembles a circle of circles. The Idea appears in each single circle, but, at the same time, the

[3] Dewey, John. *The Later Works: 1925-1953*, ed. Jo Ann Boydston.

whole Idea is constituted by the system of these peculiar phases, and each is a necessary member of the organization.[4]

So, you have wholes and then wholes and then wholes, bigger and bigger wholes. Circles of wholes and then bigger and bigger wholes. For as Mirandola states:

To divide a thing is the same as destroying it, nor can we take away from any thing its natural unity without at the same time robbing it of its integrity of being. For a whole is not its parts, but that unity which springs out of the sum of its parts, as Aristotle demonstrates in the eighth book of his Metaphysics.[5]

And now here, from a completely different field, is T. S. Eliot:

No poet, no artist of any art, has his complete meaning alone. His significance, his appreciation is the appreciation of his relation to the dead poets and artists. You cannot value him alone; you must set him, for contrast and comparison, among the dead. I mean this as a principle of aesthetic, not merely historical, criticism. The necessity that he shall conform, that

---

[4] Hegel, G.W.F. *Encyclopedia*, trans. by W. Wallace.
[5] Mirandola, op. cit.

he shall cohere, is not one-sided; what
happens when a new work of art is created
is something that happens simultaneously
to all the works of art which preceded it.
The existing monuments form an ideal
order among themselves, which is modified
by the introduction of the new (the really
new) work of art among them.[6]

So you can see the whole history of art, the whole history of the universe, as being a whole which is constantly being refashioned into a new whole as new wholes are created within it.

In his biography of Smuts, Keith Hancock states that his concept of holism started on his father's farm when as a small boy he discovered his kinship with the stones, plants and animals of that small universe of the farm.[7]

In his uncle's church . . . he had learnt
that the farm and its creatures and its
people and he himself all belonged to a
great universe, created and governed by
God. In his student years . . . he learnt
that science had a different story to tell.
Or was it the same story, told in a different
way? Eenheid, unity, became his philo-
sophical quest. His craving for eenheid,

6 *The Sacred Wood.*
7 Hancock, William Keith. *Smuts: Fields of Force.* Cambridge: Cambridge University Press, 1968.

*was now finding its nourishment not in
science and its philosophies, but in poetry
– in the poetry of Goethe, in the poetry of
Whitman.*

In fact, he went on to write a book about
Whitman which I have not been able to locate. In
the middle of his study of Whitman, Hancock says
Smuts made an exhilarating discovery. "Wholeness
was the stamp not only of persons, but of matter,
life, mind – of the universe and everything that it
contained."

And to quote from the South African
Dictionary of Biography:

[Smuts] *maintained that matter, life and
mind are not disparate phenomena but
manifestations of the cardinal principle of
Wholeness in a successive order extending
from inorganic beginnings to the highest
levels of spiritual activity, that is,
'holistically' bound to give rise to each
other in a definite series in the stages of
Evolution. The gist of the treatise is the
presupposition of Wholeness (Holism) as
a fundamental factor in the universe.*

Permit me now to give three more highly
relevant quotes from Smuts:

*One cannot help being struck by the way
in which the cells in an organism not only*

co-operate, but co-operate in a specific direction towards the fulfillment and maintenance of the type of the particular organism which they constitute. The impression is irresistible that cell activities are co-operative, that they are inherently or through selective development co-ordinated in a specific direction, and that the impress of the whole, which forms the organism is clearly stamped on all of the details.

And:

In some indefinable way this whole is not an artificial result of its parts; it is itself an active factor like its parts, and it appears to be in definite relation with them, influenced by them and again influencing them, and through this continuous interaction of parts and whole maintaining the moving equilibrium which is the organism.

And further:

Both matter and life consist of unit structures whose ordered grouping produces natural wholes which we call bodies or organisms. This characteristic of 'wholeness' meets us everywhere and points to something fundamental in the world. Holism is the term here coined for this fundamental feature of wholeness in the world [my emphasis]. *Its character is both general and specific or concrete, and it satisfies our double requirement for a natural evolutionary starting point.*

Wholes are not mere artificial constructions of thought; they actually exist; they point to something real in the universe, and Holism is a real operative feature, a vera causa. There is thus behind Evolution no mere vague creative impulse or Elan vital, but something quite definite and specific in its operation, and thus productive of the real concrete character of cosmic Evolution.

This is what I try to feel about a sufferer. This is what I mean by seeing him holistically. This is not just doing acupuncture on him or any other particular technique as a part of the rubric nowadays called holistic medicine. It is seeing every aspect of him as a whole. He is a whole, and all his functions within him are little wholes summating to this whole which is him within the wholeness of his existence within the wholeness of Existence. And in order to be able to help him, you have to help him to see himself within the wholeness of his existence in the wholeness of Existence.

If you want to call this philosophy, then the ultimate easing of the suffering of mankind is to help them in their hearts to know this philosophy of holism. Once they know their wholeness in the wholeness of Existence, they are at last at peace. They have gratefully accepted themselves in their existence.

Many years ago someone called me a clinical philosopher and I think that now I would agree with this. Clinical in the sense of helping and caring, and philosopher in the sense that central to my practice are the philosophers – Smuts, Hegel, Spinoza, Plato, Parmenides, Plotinus, Eckhart, Lao Tzu, Chuang Tzu, Mencius, Pelagius, Shankara, Ramakrishna, Vivekenanda, Dogen, Shinran and Zeno come immediately to mind. And there are many others – some old friends, some new. And the poets, the philosophers of the unconscious – especially Blake.

I believe the ultimate questions of philosophy are: Who am I in Existence? And Where? And Why? And to know this and to teach it is the only way to overcome the sufferer's anguish. So I am more and more drawn to philosophy and less and less attracted to medicine (which breaks wholes down into even smaller bits). And the philosophy I am drawn to more and more is the one, of course, which views things, people, in the whole. I hope that some time in the future the holistic practitioner will be well-grounded in philosophy – infinitely more so than I am with my smattering of readings here and there. It is what it has to be. It is philosophy – but not in the head – in the heart.

The Commitment Problem

At this point I would like to introduce what I call the Commitment Problem. To summarize: you ask someone to just look at a piece of paper (I use a piece of paper because it is innocuous, with little association – just a blank piece of paper) and he is unstressed. But if you now ask him to commit himself, his total self, to the piece of paper, then all of a sudden he becomes stressed. And this stress causes great negativity – either heart meridian anger, or else deeper hatred.

If you then take the piece of paper, fold it into four and ask the person to commit himself to the totality of the smaller piece of paper, the same stress will be there. But if you then unfold it and ask him to commit himself to a quarter of the piece of paper now delineated by the fold marks, there is no stress. This is because it is not the size of the totality that is important, but whether he can commit himself to the totality or not. And every time most people attempt to commit themselves to the totality, they go into one form or other of severe negativity.

Now you can see the difficulty of even trying to talk about the whole – let alone to practice it. I am asking the practitioner to look at the total person in his total setting – himself first, and then his patient. And there is great resistance to doing this because it is so often highly stressful, leading to negativity which defeats the therapeutic intention.

There is great resistance to looking at the whole of anything – including the very concept of holism, and the concept of holistic medicine. Everyone wants to break holistic medicine down into parts.

I recently received a brochure from a particular holistic medical association which requested holistic medicine practitioners to tick off from a list what modalities they employ. This is not holism. Holism is seeing the totality of the person, the whole of the person in the whole of his existence in the whole of Existence. And that is how the holistic practitioner has to see both himself and the sufferer before him. It is also how the sufferer has to be helped to see himself.

People have a great resistance to the whole, they want to analyze, not synthesize. In the same way as they want to relate to a bit of their existence, not all of it.

Underlying the commitment problem is always a circulation-sex meridian problem, cx-3. I first found this as a meridian problem with a schizophrenic woman who worked as a computer operator. She complained that the computer was driving her crazy. But we soon discovered that it was not the computer she was really complaining about, it was her mother. And this is at the root of the commitment problem. As soon as we start to commit ourselves to the other object, the other person, it becomes our mother who we believe hates us, and who is trying to kill us by driving us crazy. "Those whom the Gods would destroy, they first drive crazy."

This is why it is so difficult to even really discuss the concept of holism. People feel they have to instead fragmentize it for their own safety – lest they be driven mad by their mothers. They can only deal with a bit of her, not her whole. And yet the first whole picture we create is that of our mother. So, as always, my work comes back to our attitudes to our mothers and what we believe is their attitude to us.

You can envisage the whole any way you like. It is, of course, unenvisionable, ineffable, but it will always relate to the first whole – the mother, because everything, everyone else throughout our lives, is always the mother, our own individual mother as we perceived her at the beginning of life – as we constructed her entity, her entirety, as our first whole.

If what we felt from her was what we would predominantly now as adults call love, then we will have little problem with committing ourselves to the whole, to the whole as her. But if not, we will have great difficulty.

Of course, when we as adults refer to "the whole," we are certainly talking about more than our mothers. But how we relate to the whole now will always be determined by how we related to our mother as the whole when she was the whole world.

And if we want to understand the whole, we have to understand our relationship with our individual mothers and, even more so, their relationship with us. That is what is missing from Smuts and all the other philosophers: the concept that the whole world was, and in a way still is, our mothers.

The Whole Universe

When and where do the wholes stop merging? Smuts says that you have this whole which is, as it were, an integral necessary part of a total whole, as every cell is of the organism, as every atom as a whole is of the whole of the organism. So how far do these wholes go? Is there some point at which they cease to merge? Yes, when they are all seen as being THE WHOLE.

The physicist-philosopher David Bohm contrasted the lens with the hologram. The former is analytic, it enables us to accurately see a small – minutely small – aspect of reality. But the holographic image is markedly different – the very contrary:

> *The key new feature of this (holographic) record is that each part contains information about the whole object ... the form and structure of the entire object may be said to be enfolded within each region of the philosophic record.*[8]

---

[8] Bohm, David. *Wholeness and the Implicate Order*, New York: Routledge, 1995.

All the information of the whole is contained
– is enfolded, to use Bohm's word – in each and
every part. All the universe in every particular.
Blake, of course, knew this:

To see a World in a Grain of Sand
And a Heaven in a Wild Flower,
Hold Infinity in the palm of your hand
And Eternity in an hour.

With our lens we unfold a tiny fragment of the
enfolded Whole and delude ourselves that we know
All. Blake did not use a lens. He did not examine
– he admired, he adored. He Knew the Whole.

In the last chapter of *Holism and Evolution*,
entitled "The Holistic Universe," Smuts states:

Holism has been presented in the foregoing
chapters as the ultimate synthetic ordering,
organising, regulative feature in the
universe which explains all the structural
groupings and syntheses in it, from the
atom and the physico-chemical structures,
through the cell and organisms, through
Mind in animals, to Personality in man.
The all-pervading and ever-increasing
character of synthetic unity or wholeness
in these structures leads to the concept of
Holism as fundamental, and to the view of
the universe as a Holistic Universe.

To again quote Smuts:

*As we enlarge each whole, the field of each whole, we get into bigger wholes in the same way that trees become forests until we expand into the total whole, into the one. You see **oneness is just another word for the whole*** [my emphasis].

And further:

It is as if the Great Creative Spirit hath said: "Behold, I make all things whole."

And it is just a small further step from "Behold, I make all things whole" to declare "All is one Whole" and then "All is One." There is, proclaims Smuts, a force in Nature to construct wholes, all summating to The Whole. It is the nature of Nature to be whole. Nature is whole. There is only The Whole. The Whole – The One.

The great Greek scholar F. M. Cornford comments on Parmenides:

This One Being is not a mere abstraction; it proves to be a single continuous and homogenous substance filling the whole of space.[9]

Consider this *Encyclopedia Britannica* statement on Parmenides:

---

[9] Cornford, F.M. *Plato & Parmenides*. London: 1939.

Parmenides held that the multiplicity of existing things, their changing forms and motion, are but an appearance of a single eternal reality ("being"), thus giving rise to the Parmenidian principle "all is one."

All is The One. What the Vedantists call Brahman. You can call it the Absolute which, after all, Sri Aurobindo did. I'm going to use the word Brahman because I wish to mention some aspects of Vedanta philosophy.

Here are some "definitions" of Brahman (as if Brahman can be defined!): the impersonal, imperishable, absolute Existence. The Godhead. The all-pervading transcendental Reality. The Absolute.

And now from Shankara (788–820 A.D.):

From the standpoint of the illuminated soul, Brahman fills everything – beginningless, endless, immeasurable, unchanging, one without a second. In Brahman there is no diversity whatsoever. Brahman is pure existence, pure consciousness, eternal bliss, beyond action. Brahman is the innermost consciousness, filled full of endless bliss, infinite, omnipresent. Brahman cannot be avoided since it is everywhere. Brahman cannot be grasped since it is transcendent. It cannot be contained, since it contains all things.

Brahman is without parts or attributes. It is subtle, absolute taintless. Brahman is indefinable, beyond the range of mind and speech. Brahman is reality; itself established in its glory; pure, absolute consciousness, having no equal, one without a second. In Brahman there is no diversity whatsoever.[10]

In most religions there is a basic dualism between God and the individual. God is up there – and I am down here. I am not God, God is not me. These are called the dualistic schools. Judeo-Christianity is very much a dualistic school. The Shankara school is the opposite – non-dualistic or monistic. Hence, "Brahman is a concept that has no equivalent in the religions of dualism."[11]

The eternal principle within each individual the Vedantists call *atman*. The individual soul is atman within the universal soul, Brahman. Brahman – God, atman – the self. And Brahman is atman, atman is Brahman.

In *The Encyclopedia of Eastern Philosophy and Religion*, we find this statement about Advaita-Vedanta:

Its most important representative is Shankara. Advaita-Vedanta teaches that

---

[10] *Crest-Jewel of Discrimination*, trans. by Swami Prabhavananda and Christopher Isherwood. Hollywood: Vedanta Press, 1947.
[11] Ibid.

*the manifest creation, the soul, and God
are identical. Just as particle physicists
have discovered that matter consists of
continually moving fields of energy, so the
sages of Vedanta recognized that reality
consists of energy in the form of
consciousness and that human beings
perceive a gross universe by means of
gross senses, because of identification
with the ego-limited body. That which is
real and unchanging is superimposed in
the mind by the notion of an ever-changing
manifest world of names and shapes.*[12]

It is only because of our misprocessing, our
maya, our illusion, that we don't see that we as
atman are all one with Brahman.

*Shankara's best-known example is the
piece of rope that in the dark is taken
for a snake. Anxiety, repugnance, heart
palpitations are induced by a snake that
was never born and never will die, but
exists only in one's mind. Once the rope is
recognized under light as a rope, it cannot
turn back into a snake. The initial error
involves not only nescience of what is, but
also the superimposition of a notion that
has nothing to do with what is.*[13]

---

[12] Boston: Shambala, 1994.
[13] Ibid.

Advaita-Vedanta teaches that we in our ignorance continually impose the idea of snake, the manifest world, on the rope, on Brahman. Freed from illusion, Shankara declares:

May this one sentence proclaim the essence of a thousand books: Brahman alone is real, the self is nothing but Brahman.

We all are Brahman, we all are the Whole, we all are one, we all are The One.

Shankara wasn't alone in saying this – he came out of this whole school of Advaita-Vedanta of which he was a major exponent.

It also occurred in the West. Probably the best example is Spinoza who believed that "reality cannot be divided into a part which is 'God' and a part which is not-God."[14] To Spinoza, there cannot be any not-God:

In natural theology, Spinoza in Ethics breaks with Judaeo-Christian orthodoxy by conceiving God, not as the creator of human beings and of the world they inhabit, but as an infinite being 'in' which they exist as finite modes. No substance except God he contends, can be, or be conceived; and he draws the inevitable inference that the extended and thinking things of everyday experience 'are either attributes of God or

14 Armstrong, Karen. *A History of God.* New York: Ballentine Books, 1993.

affections, that is modes of God's attributes.'
God, he concludes, cannot create anything
outside himself.[15]

That is to say that God creates everything, therefore *we all are one with the One.* I believe this is the only way that we can truly find peace on earth – to realize that we are one with the One. And the one is at first our mother – and later whatever construct, whatever concept, we superimpose on her.

Holism and Health

Disease is the turning inward into the self whereas health is the reaching out selflessly to the other. Disease is egoism – health is altruism.

It has been said that at the time you reach out in altruism you are one with the other. It is more than that. Real altruism is when you and the other are one with the One – that there is no other. Thus, in a sense, the word *altruism* was a contradiction because it was derived by Comte from the Latin word *alter*, other, yet the state is achieved through oneness, the breaking down of the barrier between you and the other.

It is very easy to feel one with something which is obviously beautiful, as Blake describes in his poem "To My Friend Butts I Write My First Vision of Light."[16] And most of the experiences that led

[15] *The Cambridge Companion to Spinoza*, ed. Don Garrett. Cambridge: Cambridge University Press, 1995.

[16] Diamond, John. *The Healing Power of Blake: A Distillation.* Bloomingdale: Creativity Press, 1999.

to what the psychiatrist Richard Bucke called cosmic consciousness came from feeling one with the beautiful.

It is relatively easy to be at least superficially one with the sunset. But what about the ugly, the deformed, the decaying, the dying? Not just to feel one with that sufferer, but to kiss the leper as St. Francis did, realizing that through my oneness with him, we all are the same one. There is no other one, there is just the One. There is only the whole – and our individual wholes, so called, are just part of the total Whole.

And that is what I believe holistic healing must be. Remember Smuts knew his etymology. The word *holistic* comes from the Indo-European root *kailo*, from which are also derived *heal, whole, holy, hallow, hale* and *hearty*. They all have the same origin – and in our unconscious they are all still related.

To have health is to have a sense of wholeness and to have reverence for the wholeness as holy. So health is when you conceive of the holy holism. Only when we realize that we are this whole, and we are this One and this One is holy, only then can we have health. Now if you can in your heart understand what I just said, and if I could too, we would be in a state, I believe, of perfect health in the true sense of the word.

Healing is the embracing in the heart of the holy oneness of the holy wholeness of our Existence *just as it is*. Of the As Is.

It cannot be anything else. This is how it is. This is the As Is. This is our existence in Existence. So if we can just see that we are the whole of the wholeness and that we all are one, that there is only the One.

There seems to me to be four stages of evolution as a healer:

1. Soul to soul. To relate my soul, the divinity within me, that is me, to the divinity within the sufferer, that is the sufferer, and encouraging him to do the same back to me and to the world – especially his mother.

2. To know that my soul relates to the sufferer's soul through what Emerson called the Over-soul.

3. We are all one soul – the Over-soul. My soul is no different from yours. We are one through the Over-soul.

4. And finally: All One.

My work as a holistic healer is to try to practice this myself: to arrive at the heart knowledge from what is now book knowledge, and somehow to teach it and encourage it. I try to see the wholeness of me in the whole. All of my wholeness, the space-time, the events of my wholeness, my existence in Existence – and then to see the sufferer's existence in Existence. And then to help him to see the same, and to realize that existence is the same for all of us.

If you are to believe in holism, you have to believe that all is the Whole, all is the Holy, all is the Holy Whole, all is Existence, all is the Absolute One, all is One. You have to, in your heart, come to this understanding yourself and, by whatever means you use, encourage the sufferer to come to the same understanding. In a strange way, by very non-academic means, in a non-academic setting, you are trying to teach a form of philosophy. A philosophy, not of the mind but of the heart – the heart in the heart. And it all comes down to *All One*.

Holistic practice, no matter what you may apparently do, in the end comes down to the exhortation and encouragement, the teaching (and the example-setting) of non-dualistic philosophy.

My thanks to all the philosophers I have read who have exhorted and encouraged me with this brain knowledge which I hope will become heart Knowledge – and my mother.

Now would it be right to sum up by saying that if unity is not, nothing is?

It certainly would.[17]

---

[17] Plato. *Parmenides*, trans. by R.E. Allen. New Haven: Yale University Press, 1997.

Beyond Orion's Belt

The holistic healer
sees all of himself
as one
and all of the sufferer
as one too.
And both of them together
as one,
and that one
as part of the One.

Until I first came to America I had never seen the northern sky. In Australia I was quite able to identify the constellations, but in America I couldn't. I searched and searched for Orion's belt, and in the end it was pointed out to me. After that I was able to find it easily.

Of course, there is no Orion's belt in the sky, only a mere handful of all the visible stars that are thought to bear an imagined resemblance to the belt of the mythological Orion, once it is pointed out to us.

But there is no more relationship between the stars comprising the belt than there are between all the stars in the universe. The only relationship is that which we have created in our own fantasy.

The Universe Within

A medical diagnosis is like Orion's belt. It doesn't really exist. It is just putting together a few easily observed findings that seem to have some special relationship. But when we do this, we ignore all the thousands of other findings that are really just as equally related and equally important in the whole universe of the patient.

Each patient is a universe, and a true understanding of him is an understanding of each star in that universe and of the relationship between each star and all the other stars that comprise his universe. Not just picking a few of the stars because they make a convenient story. A true understanding of a patient is an understanding of his total universe.

This is holistic healing. It is not a number of specialists each working on a patient's individual stars, but one doctor who at all times works with an understanding and appreciation of the individuality of each star and, at the same time, the myriad inter-relationships of all the stars of the patient's universe. This is true holistic healing.

The Potter

Let's change our analogy. A potter is throwing a pot. While it is spinning on the wheel he is constantly feeling and examining it, using all of his aesthetic, artistic and intuitive faculties as well as his logical faculties. Using thus his whole creative self, he works with and molds the clay keeping it as symmetrical as possible.

Should there be one area which starts to become asymmetrical, he proceeds to rebalance and re-center this area, but he never works on only that area but always on the whole pot spinning on the wheel. Always working on the whole pot: his hands going up and down over the whole pot but concentrating most on the particular area that requires his immediate attention to restore the balance. He doesn't give that particular area a special name. He doesn't feel that there is a specific problem with that part of the pot or that separate work must be done there. He just sees that in the overall dynamic structure, which is that revolving pot on the wheel, there is one area more than the others that requires his particular attention to center it. But he always works on the whole pot.

And when the whole pot has been re-centered, he then looks again at it rotating on the wheel. Now all of his brain, his intuitive brain and his logical brain, recognizes that symmetry has been restored. And now he proceeds to work on it again, and he keeps on working until such time as he feels that the form that he envisaged has been achieved and that the pot is balanced and centered and perfect in every way. When this point is reached, his artistic needs are satisfied, and he now feels that the pot is ready to leave him, to go out into the world on its own – balanced, centered, a thing of beauty, an aspiration to Heaven and an inspiration to Earth. By its very presence, reminding us of all that is perfect and balanced and peaceful and calm and loving in our existence.

So it is with a patient. When the doctor works in a holistic fashion with him, he is all the time working with all of him, certainly concentrating a little more here where it is needed at that time – this will change from visit to visit, even from moment to moment – but always being conscious of the whole and always being aware that the part that most requires immediate correction, the part that the patient most wants corrected, is but one small tiny portion of the whole and will be corrected only when the whole is corrected and balanced.

And so he keeps doing this, session by session. Re-balancing and re-centering, until the patient and the doctor both feel that he is now ready to go out into the world on his own. He has been centered as best as possible, strengthened as far as possible against the buffets of the world. He is now ready to go out as a therapeutic communication to the world, spreading his peace, his balance and calmness and joy and love to all. The balanced, centered, integrated creature that exists inside each of us.

But remember that whenever the potter concentrates exclusively on one part of the rotating pot, which he feels requires more attention, the integrity of the whole structure will be destroyed. He can shape and create symmetry and perfection only when he is always working up and down and around the whole structure. That is my understanding of holistic medicine.

The Wise Astronomer

Forget the medical diagnosis. It is only a name. It is only an Orion's belt in the whole firmament of the universe of the patient. The doctor must breach the narrow confines that most institutions want him to work within. He must think of the totality of the patient. To see him as anything less, to reduce his existence to a diagnosis, is an insult. To see him in his totality is to worship him as a Being.

Holistic medicine really implies the absence of using any diagnostic label. The best label is the name of the patient, because we each suffer from the disease which is our selves. The diagnostic label for John Smith is "John Smith."

The holistic doctor must remember that the patient is, at this moment in time when we see him, at the end point of all the shaping forces that have influenced him throughout his existence. He is at this moment the sum total of his genetic endowment, of the nutritional status of his parents and of himself, of their emotional states and desires, and of his own. He is the culmination of all the shaping social forces that have acted on him and his family up until this minute.

When the holistic doctor observes the firmament of the sky that is the patient, he is seeing an instantaneous picture of all the end points, of all the shapings, the ebbs and flows of the universe since the beginning of time that create that picture. He knows that in the next instant, and in every instant after that, the picture will change and will continue to change with all the shaping forces of the universe.

So when he looks at a patient, he must remember that he is seeing him as the end product of all that has been and realize that this will change in the future just as surely as it has changed in the past and developed into that which he sees now.

This is the only way that we can ever think of any patient. And we aspire that, with our help, the patient's universe may be somewhat more luminous and harmonious.

———

Reprise

You can only really think holistically, embrace holism – know in your heart that you are one with The One, that atman is Brahman – when you have found at last your basic Identity.

That is to say you can only truly surrender your self when you know who your real self is, your deepest Self.

And this, your basic Identity, is always that I am Love – because I am the object of Love. I am the Beloved – of the Universe, of my mother, my first universe, as the Universe.

And All is Love. There is only ever Love. The whole Universe is Love.

> *For I think it is Love,*
> *For I feel it is Love,*
> *For I'm sure it is nothing but Love!*
> LEWIS CARROLL

To Know the Universe as Love you must first so Know your mother.

The whole Universe, the Holistic Universe, is Love – because so was, and is, my mother.

For I think she is Love,
For I feel she is Love,
For I Know she is nothing but Love!

———

John Diamond, M.D.

John Diamond, M.D., D.P.M., F.R.A.N.Z.C.P., M.R.C. Psych., F.I.A.P.M., D.I.B.A.K., specialized in psychiatry and then in holistic medicine. He is a Fellow of the Royal Australian and New Zealand College of Psychiatry, a Foundation Member of the Royal College of Psychiatrists, a Member of the American Holistic Medical Association, a Diplomate of the International Board of Applied Kinesiology and is a Fellow and past President of the International Academy of Preventive Medicine. He has held numerous senior clinical and university teaching appointments in clinical psychiatry, basic sciences and the humanities, has lectured extensively throughout the world and is a best-selling author.

As a Holistic Consultant, Dr. Diamond is concerned with all aspects of the totality of the sufferer, how they relate and how all must be involved in every healing process. His over forty years of research and practice in medicine, psychiatry, complementary medicine and holistic healing have led him to investigate many modalities which affect body, mind and spirit.

In his teaching, writing, lectures and private practice he draws on insights from all of his experience to provide guidelines for holistic living. His approach combines the idealistic and the practical, supplying tools each individual can use in all aspects of life, both professional and personal.

For more information, please contact:

The Diamond Center
PO Box 381
South Salem, NY 10590 USA
(914) 533-2158

mail@diamondcenter.net
www.diamondcenter.net